Contents

INTRODUCTION

Cannabis sativa, reefer, reggie, weed, pot, herb, trees, ganja, green, loud, marijuana, or medicine. However you refer to it, weed combined with butter is much like liquid gold. For centuries, people have consumed cannabis-infused foods to assist withailments like pain, lack of appetite, or simply to chill out. The potency of the weed butter you make is up to you. It can be powerful enough to ease chronic pain yet mild enough to allow a gentle mellowness to spread throughout the body and mind—sometimes needed after a stressful day. This versatility is what makes weed butter so great and why I'm here to help you along the way. Ingesting cannabis as food turns out to be better for your health, especially for those concerned with the effects of smoking. Although the jury is still out on whether resin and smoke from cannabis is responsible for chronic illness, weed butters and oils are the perfect alternative for anyone prudent who prefers to avoid the health side effects (and occasional social stigmas) of smoking weed.

Whether you're adding cannabis-infused butter (also known as cannabutter) into cookies, toast, or boxed macaroni and cheese, it's a multi-use miracle.

Inconspicuous and versatile, weed butter is one of the simplest ways to make an edible, and one of the least expensive ways to administer medical marijuana to a patient. Many store-bought edibles contain obscene amounts of sugars and unwanted chemicals. But when making your own cannabutter out of butter or coconut or avocado oil, it can help you recover from the symptoms of chemotherapy or anorexia without unnecessary ingredients that are not suitable for certain patients. And still others can choose to add a recreational drizzle of weed olive oil onto avocado toast for a relaxing Saturday morning. The ways to implement weed butter or oils into your meals are as infinite as the foods we eat.

CHAPTER ONE

<u>Cannabis</u>

Cannabis, also known as marijuana (Spanish pronunciation: [maɾiˈwana]) among other names,[a] is a psychoactive drug from the Cannabis plant used primarily for medical or recreational purposes. The main psychoactive component of cannabis is tetrahydrocannabinol (THC), which is one of the 483 known compounds in the plant, including at least 65 other cannabinoids, including cannabidiol (CBD). Cannabis can be used by smoking, vaporizing, within food, or as an extract.

Cannabis has various mental and physical effects, which include euphoria, altered states of mind and sense of time, difficulty concentrating, impaired short-term memory and body movement, relaxation, and an increase in appetite. Onset of effects is felt within minutes when smoked, and about 30 to 60 minutes when cooked and eaten.The effects last for two to six hours, depending on the amount used. At high doses, mental effects can include anxiety, delusions (including ideas of reference), hallucinations, panic, paranoia, and psychosis. There is a strong relation between cannabis use and the risk of psychosis,though the direction of causality is debated.Physical effects include increased heart rate, difficulty breathing, nausea, and behavioral problems in children whose mothers used cannabis during pregnancy;short-term side effects may also include dry mouth and red eyes.Long-term adverse effects may include addiction, decreased mental ability in those who started regular use as adolescents, chronic coughing, and susceptibility to respiratory infections.

Cannabis is mostly used recreationally or as a medicinal drug, although it may also be used for spiritual purposes. In 2013, between 128 and 232 million people used cannabis (2.7% to 4.9% of the global population between the ages of 15 and 65). It is one of the most commonly used drugs in the world, and used both legally and illegally, with the highest use among adults (as of 2018) in Zambia, the United States, Canada, and Nigeria. While cannabis plants have been grown since at least the 3rd millennium BCE,evidence suggests that it was being smoked for psychoactive effects at least 2,500 years ago in the Pamir Mountains;the earliest evidence found at a cemetery in what is today western China close to the tripoint with Tajikistan and Afghanistan. Since the early 20th century, cannabis has been subject to legal restrictions. The possession, use, and cultivation of cannabis is illegal in most countries of the world.

In 2013, Uruguay became the first country to legalize recreational use of cannabis.Other countries to do so are Canada, Georgia, and South Africa, along with 11 states and the District of Columbia in the United States (though the drug remains federally illegal). Medical use of cannabis, requiring the approval of a physician, has been legalized in many countries

Uses Of Cannabis

Medical

Medical cannabis, or medical marijuana, can refer to the use of cannabis and its cannabinoids to treat disease or improve symptoms; however, there is no single agreed-upon definition. The rigorous scientific study of cannabis as a medicine has been hampered by production restrictions and by the fact that it is classified as an illegal drug by many governments. There is limited evidence suggesting cannabis can be used to reduce nausea and vomiting during chemotherapy, to improve appetite in people with HIV/AIDS, or to treat chronic pain and muscle spasms. Its use for other medical applications is insufficient for drawing conclusions about safety or efficacy.

Short-term use increases the risk of both minor and major adverse effects. Common side effects include dizziness, feeling tired and vomiting. The long-term effects of cannabis are not clear. There are concerns surrounding memory and cognition problems, risk of addiction, risk of schizophrenia in young people, and the risk of children taking it by accident.

Cannabis has psychoactive and physiological effects when consumed. The immediate desired effects from consuming cannabis include relaxation and euphoria (the "high" or "stoned" feeling), a general alteration of conscious perception, increased awareness of sensation, increased libido and distortions in the perception of time and space. At higher doses, effects can include altered body image, auditory and/or visual illusions, pseudohallucinations and ataxia from selective impairment of polysynaptic reflexes. [citation needed] In some cases, cannabis can lead to dissociative states such as depersonalization and derealization.

Some immediate undesired side effects include a decrease in short-term memory, dry mouth, impaired motor skills and reddening of the eyes. Aside from a subjective change in perception and mood, the most common short-term physical and neurological effects include increased heart rate, increased appetite and consumption of food, lowered blood pressure, impairment of short-term and working memory, psychomotor coordination, and concentration. Some users may experience an episode of acute psychosis, which usually abates after six hours, but in rare instances, heavy users may find the symptoms continuing for many days.

A reduced quality of life is associated with heavy cannabis use, although the relationship is inconsistent and weaker than for tobacco and other substances. The direction of cause and effect, however, is unclear.

Cannabis has held sacred status in several religions and has served as an entheogen – a chemical substance used in religious, shamanic, or spiritual contexts– in the Indian subcontinent since the Vedic period dating back to approximately 1500 BCE, but perhaps as far back as 2000 BCE. There are several references in Greek mythology to a powerful drug that eliminated anguish and sorrow. Herodotus wrote about early ceremonial practices by the Scythians, thought to have occurred from the 5th to 2nd century BCE. In modern culture, the spiritual use of cannabis has been spread by the disciples of the Rastafari movement who use cannabis as a sacrament and as an aid to meditation. The earliest known reports regarding the sacred status of cannabis in the Indian subcontinent come from the Atharva Veda, estimated to have been composed sometime around 1400 BCE.

Available forms

Cannabis is consumed in many different ways, all of which involve heating to decarboxylate THCA in the plant into THC.

• Smoking, which typically involves burning and inhaling vaporized cannabinoids ("smoke") from small pipes, bongs (portable versions of hookahs with a water chamber), paper-wrapped joints or tobacco-leaf-wrapped blunts, and other items.

• Vaporizer, which heats any form of cannabis to 165–190 °C (329–374 °F),causing the active ingredients to evaporate into vapor without burning the plant material (the boiling point of THC is 157 °C (315 °F) at atmospheric pressure).

• Cannabis tea, which contains relatively small concentrations of THC because THC is an oil (lipophilic) and is only slightly water-soluble (with a solubility of 2.8 mg per liter). Cannabis tea is made by first adding a saturated fat to hot water (e.g. cream or any milk except skim) with a small amount of cannabis.

• Edibles, where cannabis is added as an ingredient to one of a variety of foods, including butter and baked goods. In India it is commonly made into a beverage, bhang.

• Capsules, typically containing cannabis oil, and other dietary supplement products, for which some 220 were approved in Canada in 2018.

Adverse Effect

Short term

Acute effects may include anxiety and panic, impaired attention and memory, an increased risk of psychotic symptoms, the inability to think clearly, and an increased risk of accidents.Cannabis impairs a person's driving ability, and THC was the illicit drug most frequently found in the blood of drivers who have been involved in vehicle crashes. Those with THC in their system are from three to seven times more likely to be the cause of the accident than those who had not used either cannabis or alcohol, although its role is not necessarily causal because THC stays in the bloodstream for days to weeks after intoxication.

According to the United States Department of Health and Human Services, there were 455,000 emergency room visits associated with cannabis use in 2011. These statistics include visits in which the patient was treated for a condition induced by or related to recent cannabis use. The drug use must be "implicated" in the emergency department visit, but does not need to be the direct cause of the visit. Most of the illicit drug emergency room visits involved multiple drugs.In 129,000 cases, cannabis was the only implicated drug.

The short term effects of cannabis can be altered if it has been laced with opioid drugs such as heroin or fentanyl.The added drugs are meant to enhance the psychoactive properties, add to its weight, and increase profitability, despite the increased danger of overdose.

Long term

Heavy, long-term exposure to marijuana may have biologically based physical, mental, behavioral and social health consequences and may be "associated with diseases of the liver (particularly with co-existing hepatitis C), lungs, heart, and vasculature". Mothers who used marijuana during pregnancy have children with more depression, hyperactivity, and inattention. It is recommended that cannabis use be stopped before and during pregnancy as it can result in negative outcomes for both the mother and baby.

However, maternal use of marijuana during pregnancy does not appear to be associated with low birth weight or early delivery after controlling for tobacco use and other confounding factors.

A 2014 review found that while cannabis use may be less harmful than alcohol use, the recommendation to substitute it for problematic drinking was premature without further study.Various surveys conducted between 2015 and 2019 found that many users of cannabis substitute it for prescription drugs (including opioids), alcohol, and tobacco; most of those who used it in place of alcohol or tobacco either reduced or stopped their intake of the latter substances.

A limited number of studies have examined the effects of cannabis smoking on the respiratory system.Chronic heavy marijuana smoking is associated with coughing, production of sputum, wheezing, and other symptoms of chronic bronchitis. The available evidence does not support a causal relationship between cannabis use and chronic obstructive pulmonary disease.Short-term use of cannabis is associated with bronchodilation.Other side effects of cannabis use include cannabinoid hyperemesis syndrome (CHS).

Cannabis smoke contains thousands of organic and inorganic chemical compounds. This tar is chemically similar to that found in tobacco smoke, and over fifty known carcinogens have been identified in cannabis smoke,including; nitrosamines, reactive aldehydes, and polycylic hydrocarbons, including benz[a]pyrene. Cannabis smoke is also inhaled more deeply than tobacco smoke.

As of 2015, there is no consensus regarding whether cannabis smoking is associated with an increased risk of cancer. Light and moderate use of cannabis is not believed to increase risk of lung or upper airway cancer. Evidence for causing these cancers is mixed concerning heavy, long-term use.

In general, there are far lower risks of pulmonary complications for regular cannabis smokers when compared with those of tobacco.

A 2015 review found an association between cannabis use and the development of testicular germ cell tumors (TGCTs), particularly non-seminoma TGCTs. Another 2015 meta-analysis found no association between lifetime cannabis use and risk of head or neck cancer.Combustion products are not present when using a vaporizer, consuming THC in pill form, or consuming cannabis foods.

There is concern that cannabis may contribute to cardiovascular disease, but as of 2018, evidence of this relationship was unclear. Research in these events is complicated because cannabis is often used in conjunction with tobacco, and drugs such as alcohol and cocaine. Smoking cannabis has also been shown to increase the risk of myocardial infarction by 4.8 times for the 60 minutes after consumption.

Neuroimaging

Although global abnormalities in white matter and grey matter are not associated with cannabis abuse, reduced hippocampal volume is consistently found. Amygdala abnormalities are sometimes reported, although findings are inconsistent.

Cannabis use is associated with increased recruitment of task-related areas, such as the dorsolateral prefrontal cortex, which is thought to reflect compensatory activity due to reduced processing efficiency.Cannabis use is also associated with downregulation of CB1 receptors. The magnitude of down regulation is associated with cumulative cannabis exposure, and is reversed after one month of abstinence. There is limited evidence that chronic cannabis use can reduce levels of glutamate metabolites in the human brain.

Cognition

A 2015 meta analysis found that, although a longer period of abstinence was associated with smaller magnitudes of impairment, both retrospective and prospective memory were impaired in cannabis users. The authors concluded that some, but not all, of the deficits associated with cannabis use were reversible. A 2012 meta analysis found that deficits in most domains of cognition persisted beyond the acute period of intoxication, but was not evident in studies where subjects were abstinent for more than 25 days.Few high quality studies have been performed on the long-term effects of cannabis on cognition, and the results were generally inconsistent.

Furthermore, effect sizes of significant findings were generally small. One review concluded that, although most cognitive faculties were unimpaired by cannabis use, residual deficits occurred in executive functions.Impairments in executive functioning are most consistently found in older populations, which may reflect heavier cannabis exposure, or developmental effects associated with adolescent cannabis use.One review found three prospective cohort studies that examined the relationship between self reported cannabis use and intelligence quotient (IQ). The study following the largest number of heavy cannabis users reported that IQ declined between ages 7–13 and age 38. Poorer school performance and increased incidence of leaving school early were both associated with cannabis use, although a causal relationship was not established.Cannabis users demonstrated increased activity in task-related brain regions, consistent with reduced processing efficiency.

Psychiatric

At an epidemiological level, a dose–response relationship exists between cannabis use and increased risk of psychosis and earlier onset of psychosis.

Although the epidemiological association is robust, evidence to prove a causal relationship is lacking.But a biological causal pathway is plausible, especially if there is a genetic predisposition to mental illness, in which case cannabis may be a trigger.

It is not clear whether cannabis use affects the rate of suicide. Cannabis may also increase the risk of depression, but insufficient research has been performed to draw a conclusion.Cannabis use is associated with increased risk of anxiety disorders, although causality has not been established.

A February 2019 review found that cannabis use during adolescence was associated with an increased risk of developing depression and suicidal behavior later in life, while finding no effect on anxiety.

Reinforcement disorders

About 9% of those who experiment with marijuana eventually become dependent according to DSM-IV (1994) criteria. A 2013 review estimates daily use is associated with a 10–20% rate of dependence.The highest risk of cannabis dependence is found in those with a history of poor academic achievement, deviant behavior in childhood and adolescence, rebelliousness, poor parental relationships, or a parental history of drug and alcohol problems. Of daily users, about 50% experience withdrawal upon cessation of use (i.e. are dependent), characterized by sleep problems, irritability, dysphoria, and craving. Cannabis withdrawal is less severe than withdrawal from alcohol.

According to DSM-V criteria, 9% of those who are exposed to cannabis develop cannabis use disorder, compared to 20% for cocaine, 23% for alcohol and 68% for nicotine. Cannabis abuse disorder in the DSM-V involves a combination of DSM-IV criteria for cannabis abuse and dependence, plus the addition of craving, minus the criterion related to legal troubles.

Pharmacology

Mechanism of action

The high lipid-solubility of cannabinoids results in their persisting in the body for long periods of time. Even after a single administration of THC, detectable levels of THC can be found in the body for weeks or longer (depending on the amount administered and the sensitivity of the assessment method).Investigators have suggested that this is an important factor in marijuana's effects, perhaps because cannabinoids may accumulate in the body, particularly in the lipid membranes of neurons.

Researchers confirmed that THC exerts its most prominent effects via its actions on two types of cannabinoid receptors, the CB1 receptor and the CB2 receptor, both of which are G protein-coupled receptors.The CB1 receptor is found primarily in the brain as well as in some peripheral tissues, and the

CB2 receptor is found primarily in peripheral tissues, but is also expressed in neuroglial cells.THC appears to alter mood and cognition through its agonist actions on the CB1 receptors, which inhibit a secondary messenger system (adenylate cyclase) in a dose-dependent manner.

Via CB1 receptor activation, THC indirectly increases dopamine release and produces psychotropic effects.CBD also acts as an allosteric modulator of the μ- and δ-opioid receptors.THC also potentiates the effects of the glycine receptors. It is unknown if or how these actions contribute to the effects of cannabis

Chemistry

Detection in body fluids

THC and its major (inactive) metabolite, THC-COOH, can be measured in blood, urine, hair, oral fluid or sweat using chromatographic techniques as part of a drug use testing program or a forensic investigation of a traffic or other criminal offense.The concentrations obtained from such analyses can often be helpful in distinguishing active use from passive exposure, elapsed time since use, and extent or duration of use. These tests cannot, however, distinguish authorized cannabis smoking for medical purposes from unauthorized recreational smoking.Commercial cannabinoid immunoassays, often employed as the initial screening method when testing physiological specimens for marijuana presence, have different degrees of cross-reactivity with THC and its metabolites.Urine contains predominantly THC-COOH, while hair, oral fluid and sweat contain primarily THC.Blood may contain both substances, with the relative amounts dependent on the recency and extent of usage.

The Duquenois–Levine test is commonly used as a screening test in the field, but it cannot definitively confirm the presence of cannabis, as a large range of substances have been shown to give false positives. Researchers at John Jay College of Criminal Justice reported that dietary zinc supplements can mask the presence of THC and other drugs in urine.

 However, a 2013 study conducted by researchers at the University of Utah School of Medicine refute the possibility of self-administered zinc producing false-negative urine drug test

Varieties and Strain

CBD is a 5-HT1A receptor agonist, which is under laboratory research to determine if it has an anxiolytic effect.It is often claimed that sativa strains provide a more stimulating psychoactive high while indica strains are more sedating with a body high.

 However, this is disputed by researchers.

Psychoactive ingredients

According to the United Nations Office on Drugs and Crime (UNODC), "the amount of THC present in a cannabis sample is generally used as a measure of cannabis potency." The three main forms of cannabis products are the flower/fruit, resin (hashish), and oil (hash oil). The UNODC states that cannabis often contains 5% THC content, resin "can contain up to 20% THC content", and that "Cannabis oil may contain more than 60% THC content."

A 2012 review found that the THC content in marijuana had increased worldwide from 1970 to 2009.It is unclear, however, whether the increase in THC content has caused people to consume more THC or if users adjust based on the potency of the cannabis. It is likely that the higher THC content allows people to ingest less tar. At the same time, CBD levels in seized samples have lowered, in part because of the desire to produce higher THC levels and because more illegal growers cultivate indoors using artificial lights. This helps avoid detection but reduces the CBD production of the plant.

Australia's National Cannabis Prevention and Information Centre (NCPIC) states that the buds (infructescences) of the female cannabis plant contain the highest concentration of THC, followed by the leaves. The stalks and seeds have "much lower THC levels". The UN states that the leaves can contain ten times less THC than the buds, and the stalks one hundred times less THC.

After revisions to cannabis scheduling in the UK, the government moved cannabis back from a class C to a class B drug. A purported reason was the appearance of high potency cannabis. They believe skunk accounts for between 70 and 80% of samples seized by police (despite the fact that skunk can sometimes be incorrectly mistaken for all types of herbal cannabis). Extracts such as hashish and hash oil typically contain more THC than high potency cannabis infructescences.

Preparation

Marijuana

Marijuana or marihuana (herbal cannabis) consists of the dried flowers and fruits and subtending leaves and stems of the female Cannabis plant. This is the most widely consumed form, containing 3% to 20% THC, with reports of up to 33% THC.This is the stock material from which all other preparations are derived. Although herbal cannabis and industrial hemp derive from the same species and contain the psychoactive component (THC), they are distinct strains with unique biochemical compositions and uses. Hemp has lower concentrations of THC and higher concentrations of CBD, which gives lesser psychoactive effects.

Kief

Kief is a powder, rich in trichomes, which can be sifted from the leaves, flowers and fruits of cannabis plants and either consumed in powder form or compressed to produce cakes of hashish. The word "kif" derives from colloquial Arabic كيف kēf/kīf, meaning pleasure.

Hashish

Hashish (also spelled hasheesh, hashisha, or simply hash) is a concentrated resin cake or ball produced from pressed kief, the detached trichomes and fine material that falls off cannabis fruits, flowers and leaves. or from scraping the resin from the surface of the plants and rolling it into balls. It varies in color from black to golden brown depending upon purity and variety of cultivar it was obtained from. It can be consumed orally or smoked, and is also vaporized, or 'vaped'. The term "rosin hash" refers to a high quality solventless product obtained through heat and pressure.

Tincture

Cannabinoids can be extracted from cannabis plant matter using high-proof spirits (often grain alcohol) to create a tincture, often referred to as "green dragon".

Nabiximols is a branded product name from a tincture manufacturing pharmaceutical company.

Hash oil

Hash oil is a resinous matrix of cannabinoids obtained from the Cannabis plant by solvent extraction, formed into a hardened or viscous mass. Hash oil can be the most potent of the main cannabis products because of its high level of psychoactive compound per its volume, which can vary depending on the plant's mix of essential oils and psychoactive compounds. Butane and supercritical carbon dioxide hash oil have become popular in recent years.

Infusions

There are many varieties of cannabis infusions owing to the variety of non-volatile solvents used. The plant material is mixed with the solvent and then pressed and filtered to express the oils of the plant into the solvent. Examples of solvents used in this process are cocoa butter, dairy butter, cooking oil, glycerine, and skin moisturizers. Depending on the solvent, these may be used in cannabis foods or applied topically.

Medical use

Medical marijuana refers to the use of the Cannabis plant as a physician-recommended herbal therapy as well as synthetic THC and cannabinoids. So far, the medical use of cannabis is legal only in a limited number of territories, including Canada,Belgium, Australia, the Netherlands, New Zealand,Spain, and many U.S. states. This usage generally requires a prescription, and distribution is usually done within a framework defined by local laws. There is evidence supporting the use of cannabis or its derivatives in the treatment of chemotherapy-induced nausea and vomiting, neuropathic pain, and multiple sclerosis. Lower levels of evidence support its use for AIDS wasting syndrome, epilepsy, rheumatoid arthritis, and glaucoma

History

Ancient history

Cannabis is indigenous to Central Asia and the Indian subcontinent, and its uses for fabric and rope dates back to the Neolithic age in China and Japan.It is unclear when cannabis first became known for its psychoactive properties. The oldest archeological evidence for the burning of cannabis was found in Romanian kurgans dated 3,500 BC, and scholars suggest that the drug was first used in ritual ceremonies by Proto-Indo-European tribes living in the Pontic-Caspian steppe during the Chalcolithic period, a custom they eventually spread throughout western Eurasia during the Indo-Europan migrations. Some research suggests that the ancient Indo-Iranian drug soma, mentioned in the Vedas, sometimes contained cannabis. This is based on the discovery of a basin containing cannabis in a shrine of the second millennium BC in Turkmenistan.

Cannabis was known to the ancient Assyrians, who discovered its psychoactive properties through the Iranians. Using it in some religious ceremonies, they called it qunubu (meaning "way to produce smoke"), a probable origin of the modern word "cannabis". The Iranians also introduced cannabis to the Scythians, Thracians and Dacians, whose shamans (the kapnobatai—"those who walk on smoke/clouds") burned cannabis infructescences to induce trance. The plant was used in China before 2800 BC, and found therapeutic use in India by 1000 BC, where it was used in food and drink, including bhang.

Cannabis has an ancient history of ritual use and is found in pharmacological cults around the world. The earliest evidence of cannabis smoking has been found in the 2,500-year-old tombs of Jirzankal Cemetery in the Pamir Mountains in Western China, where cannabis residue were found in burners with charred pebbles possibly used during funeral rituals.Hemp seeds discovered by archaeologists at Pazyryk suggest early ceremonial practices like eating by the Scythians occurred during the 5th to

2nd century BC, confirming previous historical reports by Herodotus. It was used by Muslims in various Sufi orders as early as the Mamluk period, for example by the Qalandars.Smoking pipes uncovered in Ethiopia and carbon-dated to around c. AD 1320 were found to have traces of cannabis.

Modern history

Following an 1836–1840 travel in North Africa and the Middle East, French physician Jacques-Joseph Moreau wrote on the psychological effects of cannabis use; he was a member of Paris' Club des Hashischins. [citation needed] In 1842, Irish physician William Brooke O'Shaughnessy, who had studied the drug while working as a medical officer in Bengal with the East India company, brought a quantity of cannabis with him on his return to Britain, provoking renewed interest in the West. Examples of classic literature of the period featuring cannabis include Les paradis artificiels (1860) by Charles Baudelaire and The Hasheesh Eater (1857) by Fitz Hugh Ludlow.

Cannabis was criminalized in various countries beginning in the 19th century. The British colonies of Mauritius banned cannabis in 1840 over concerns on its effect on Indian indentured workers; the same occurred in British Singapore in 1870.In the United States, the first restrictions on sale of cannabis came in 1906 (in the District of Columbia).Canada criminalized cannabis in The Opium and Narcotic Drug Act, before any reports of the use of the drug in Canada, but eventually legalized its consumption for recreational and medicinal purposes in 2018.

In 1925, a compromise was made at an international conference in The Hague about the International Opium Convention that banned exportation of "Indian hemp" to countries that had prohibited its use, and requiring importing countries to issue certificates approving the importation and stating that the shipment was required "exclusively for medical or scientific purposes". It also required parties to "exercise an effective control of such a nature as to prevent the illicit international traffic in Indian hemp and especially in the resin". In the United States in 1937, the Marihuana Tax Act was passed, and prohibited the production of hemp in addition to cannabis.

In 1972, the Dutch government divided drugs into more- and less-dangerous categories, with cannabis being in the lesser category. Accordingly, possession of 30 grams (1.1 oz) or less was made a misdemeanor. Cannabis has been available for recreational use in coffee shops since 1976. Cannabis products are only sold openly in certain local "coffeeshops" and possession of up to 5 grams (0.18 oz) for personal use is decriminalized, however: the police may still confiscate it, which often happens in car checks near the border. Other types of sales and transportation are not permitted, although the general approach toward cannabis was lenient even before official decriminalization

In Uruguay, President Jose Mujica signed legislation to legalize recreational cannabis in December 2013, making Uruguay the first country in the modern era to legalize cannabis. In August 2014, Uruguay legalized growing up to six plants at home, as well as the formation of growing clubs, and a state-controlled marijuana dispensary regime.

As of 17 October 2018 when recreational use of cannabis was legalized in Canada, dietary supplements for human use and veterinary health products containing not more than 10 parts per million of THC extract were approved for marketing; Nabiximols (as Sativex) is used as a prescription drug in Canada.

The United Nations' World Drug Report stated that cannabis "was the world's most widely produced, trafficked, and consumed drug in the world in 2010", and estimated between 128 million and 238 million users globally in 2015.

Chemical Composition

The main component of cannabis is THC formed from decarboxylation of THCA. Raw leaf is not psychoactive because cannabinoids are in form of carboxylic acids. The major cannabinoid acids of raw cannabis are THCA, CBGA, CBDA, CBCA,

CBGVA, THCVA, CBDVA, CBCVA. They are precursors to cannabinoids. On decarboxylation the following major cannabinoids THC, CBD, CBD, CBC, CBCV, CBDV, CBGV, THCV are formed. On more degradation CBN is formed. Cannabis is rich in terpenes too. The most common terpene in cannabis are Myrcene, Limonene, Caryophyllene, Terpinolene, Pinene, Humulene, Ocimene, Linalool.

Economics

Production

Sinsemilla (Spanish for "without seed") is the dried, seedless (i.e. parthenocarpic) infructescences of female cannabis plants. Because THC production drops off once pollination occurs, the male plants (which produce little THC themselves) are eliminated before they shed pollen to prevent pollination, thus inducing the development of parthenocarpic fruits gathered in dense infructescences. Advanced cultivation techniques such as hydroponics, cloning, high-intensity artificial lighting, and the sea of green method are frequently employed as a response (in part) to prohibition enforcement efforts that make outdoor cultivation more risky.

"Skunk" refers to several named strains of potent cannabis, grown through selective breeding and sometimes hydroponics. It is a cross-breed of Cannabis sativa and C. indica (although other strains of this mix exist in abundance). Skunk cannabis potency ranges usually from 6% to 15% and rarely as high as 20%. The average THC level in coffee shops in the Netherlands is about 18–19%.

The average levels of THC in cannabis sold in the United States rose dramatically between the 1970s and 2000.This is disputed for various reasons, and there is little consensus as to whether this is a fact or an artifact of poor testing methodologies.

 According to Daniel Forbes writing for slate.com, the relative strength of modern strains are likely skewed because undue weight is given to much more expensive and potent, but less prevalent, samples. Some suggest that results are skewed by older testing methods that included low-THC-content plant material such as leaves in the samples, which are excluded in contemporary tests. Others believe that modern strains actually are significantly more potent than older ones.

Gateway drug

The gateway hypothesis states that cannabis use increases the probability of trying "harder" drugs. The hypothesis has been hotly debated as it is regarded by some as the primary rationale for the United States prohibition on cannabis use. A Pew

Research Center poll found that political opposition to marijuana use was significantly associated with concerns about the health effects and whether legalization would increase marijuana use by children.

Some studies state that while there is no proof for the gateway hypothesis, young cannabis users should still be considered as a risk group for intervention programs. Other findings indicate that hard drug users are likely to be poly-drug users, and that interventions must address the use of multiple drugs instead of a single hard drug. Almost two-thirds of the poly drug users in the 2009-2010 Scottish Crime and Justice Survey used cannabis.

The gateway effect may appear due to social factors involved in using any illegal drug. Because of the illegal status of cannabis, its consumers are likely to find themselves in situations allowing them to acquaint with individuals using or selling other illegal drugs. Studies have shown that alcohol and tobacco may additionally be regarded as gateway drugs;however, a more parsimonious explanation could be that cannabis is simply more readily available (and at an earlier age) than illegal hard drugs. In turn, alcohol and tobacco are typically easier to obtain at an earlier age than is cannabis (though the reverse may be true in some areas), thus leading to the "gateway sequence" in those individuals, since they are most likely to experiment with any drug offered.

A related alternative to the gateway hypothesis is the common liability to addiction (CLA) theory. It states that some individuals are, for various reasons, willing to try multiple recreational substances. The "gateway" drugs are merely those that are (usually) available at an earlier age than the harder drugs. Researchers have noted in an extensive review that it is dangerous to present the sequence of events described in gateway "theory" in causative terms as this hinders both research and intervention.

Research

Cannabis research is challenging since the plant is illegal in most countries. Research-grade samples of the drug are difficult to obtain for research purposes, unless granted under authority of national regulatory agencies, such as the US Food and Drug Administration.

There are also other difficulties in researching the effects of cannabis. Many people who smoke cannabis also smoke tobacco. This causes confounding factors, where questions arise as to whether the tobacco, the cannabis, or both that have caused a cancer. Another difficulty researchers have is in recruiting people who smoke cannabis into studies. Because cannabis is an illegal drug in many countries, people may be reluctant to take part in research, and if they do agree to take part, they may not say how much cannabis they actually smoke.

A 2015 review found that the use of high CBD-to-THC strains of cannabis showed significantly fewer positive symptoms, such as delusions and hallucinations, better cognitive function and both lower risk for developing psychosis, as well as a later age of onset of the illness, compared to cannabis with low CBD-to-THC ratios. Reviews in 2019 found that research was insufficient to determine the safety and efficacy of using cannabis to treat schizophrenia, psychosis, or other mental disorders. There is preliminary evidence that cannabis interferes with the anticoagulant properties of prescription drugs used for treating blood clots. As of 2019, the mechanisms for the anti-inflammatory and possible pain relieving effects of cannabis were not defined, and there were no governmental regulatory approvals or clinical practices for use of cannabis as a drug.

CHAPTER TWO

<u>What Is Weed Butter?</u>

Also known as cannabutter, weed butter is one of the most essential components to making edibles. Typically, edibles are made from cannabisinfusedfat, sugar, alcohol, or vegetable glycerin. The fat in butter and oils, however, is the optimal way to transfer the THC from cannabis into an infusion. Turns out, depending on the method you use, you can transfer more than just the THC to the fat, but rather a full spectrum of the chemical components of cannabis. This includes the nonpsychoactive properties of THCA, which quietly benefit our health. THCA is similar to CBD, the stuff that doesn't get you high. Here's the thing about fat—it's not actually that bad for you. We need fats, and it's impossible to truly have a healthy diet without them. They keep our skin supple and our hearts functioning better. Think of avocados, fatty oils from fish, and coconut oil. Fat is not only a healthy part of the human diet, but is scientifically the most efficient and most versatile way to infuse weed. But not all

fats are the same. Man-made and genetically modified fats like polyunsaturated fatty acids, monounsaturated fats, and trans fats—found in potato chips and fast food—are the culprits behind many health issues. This is mainly because they are foreign to our bodies. And though they can be found in nature, they are usually in very minute traces, which cause little harm. All in all, it's a good idea to use a natural fat, butter, or oil when infusing weed. It should also be said that not all infusion processes are the same. Different methods result in different quantities of oil or butter due to the ingredients used. Because butter cooks down more than say, coconut oil, you will be left with a bit less material. Though weed and a fatty substance is all you essentially need, some infusion methods also require a slow cooker, a stovetop, or a binder (the element used to help the weed stick to the

substance) such as grain alcohol or protein. Don't get stressed, though, I will take you through each method, step by step. It's not only easier than you think, but having these skills in the kitchen is invaluable and can also be used for just about any herb you might want to infuse. Think rosemary and cannabis-infused butter. From there, you can choose which method, which fat, and which type of weed works best for your lifestyle, given the materials and ingredients you already have on hand.

After infusing, you will be left with weed butter, allowing you to easily incorporate weed to any recipe that requires a little bit of fat. Are you one of those millennial coffee freaks who likes to add a pad of butter to your coffee in the morning? Try it with weed butter. Coffee and a small dose of cannabis (especially CBD) is becoming a popular health tool for sustaining focus throughout the day. Do you like coconut oil in your beans and rice, eggs, or soups? Try some with infused weed. Once you realize how easy it is to make weed butter, you can add it into any meal of your choice—and you'll never want to eat anything without it. The best part about making your own weed butter and edibles is that the potency is up to your personal choice and preference. One pot brownie doesn't have to send you to outer space (unless you're in that kind of mood). Meals prepared with love with the weed butter you'll make from this book can be just enough to help with anxiety or an evening of nightmares from PTSD. The edibles game has completely changed. It's more diverse and healthier than ever before.

Medical Cannabis

Medical cannabis administered in the form of edibles is by and large considered one of the best alternatives to expensive, overprescribed, and highly addictive pain medications. "Medical marijuana has been shown to be an effective treatment for pain that may also reduce the chance of opioid dependence," said Dr. Howard Zucker, the New York State Health Commissioner. "Adding opioid replacement as a qualifying condition for medical marijuana offers providers another treatment option, which is a critical step in combating the deadly opioid epidemic affecting people across the state."

According to the American Nurses Association, all types of marijuana, including cannabinoids such as THC, CBD, CBN, THCA, and others, have been widely used medically to treat certain diseases and/or suppress symptoms. "It has been used for alleviating symptoms of nausea and

vomiting; stimulating appetite in HIV patients; alleviating chronic pain;

easing spasticity due to multiple sclerosis; decreasing symptoms of depression, anxiety, sleep disorders and psychosis; and relieving intraocular pressure from glaucoma." This means that something as simple and delicious as a weed pancake or salad with infused olive oil can provide just as much or more pain relief as an expensive prescribed drug.

As the positive benefits of cannabis begin to swell into common, mainstream knowledge, and as we learn that these benefits outweigh the risks (are there any risks other than extreme munchies and sleepiness?), we see more headway in academic studies. Many labs are increasing their research in this area. In June 2018, the United Nations Drug Committee had its first ever meeting to address, analyze, and discuss the safety and health benefits of cannabis. Here's what they found: Cannabis is a "relatively safe drug"8 that millions of people have already been using globally to help manage a wide range of medical conditions.

Potency Chart

More than just a trend, microdosing and low dosing are an integral part of my personal philosophy when smoking, vaping, or eating edibles. I like to keep my THC serving sizes low. What's the point of making tasty edibles if you can't eat every last crumb? Eating in lower doses allows you to enjoy a full meal without feeling uncomfortably high. Each cannabis oil recipe in this book starts with either 7 grams (¼ ounce) or 14 grams (½ ounce) of weed. This loosely translates into about 15 mg or 30 mg of THC, respectively, for each teaspoon of oil or butter used in the entire dish.

When testing for potency, remember that it will take some time for you to feel the effects and benefits of your cannabutter, canna-oil, or cannabisinfused food. When you eat an edible, unlike when you smoke a joint, the cannabis enters your bloodstream through your gut. This means that the THC or CBD gets absorbed at a slower rate than it does when smoking or vaping. Sometimes you might feel a more intense body high. As a rule, of thumb, wait one to two hours to see how you feel before eating a second serving of your medicated meal. Try to do this on a day when you're able to chill out, in case you find that you've gotten too stoned.

Below is a handy chart to use when deciding on the potency of your weed butter. In this book, all recipes use the lowest dose, meaning that for every cup of weed butter or weed oil, there will be 700 mg of THC. Remember that 1 cup = 8 ounces = 48 teaspoons. If you've had a serving and don't feel anything after two hours, it's okay to try some more.

Weed Butter Potency

Dose

Low dose

Quantity of weed, before infusion

¼ ounce (7g)

%THC/strain

10 percent

Infused butter, oil, or fat

1 cup/2 sticks

THC or CBD/cup

700 mg

THC or CBD (mg)/teaspoon

14.58

Dose

Moderate dose

Quantity of weed, before infusion

½ ounce (14g)

%THC/strain

10 percent

Infused butter, oil, or fat

1 cup/2 sticks

THC or CBD/cup

1400 mg

THC or CBD (mg)/teaspoon

29.17

Dose

Potent dose

Quantity of weed, before infusion

1 ounce (28g)

%THC/strain

10 percent

Infused butter, oil, or fat

1 cup/2 sticks

THC or CBD/cup

2800 mg

THC or CBD (mg)/teaspoon

53.33

The average strain of marijuana will contain approximately 10 percent of THC. However, different strains may have different percentages of THC and/or CBD. Take note of the labels on weed purchased from a dispensary or retailer, which should list the percentage. If they do not, find out the name or strain—it's always a good idea to know which strain you are using. If you know the name of your weed, you can easily look it up online. I know, the internet, right? On a secure device, simply search for the strain followed by "percentage of THC." Leafly.com is a great resource for this. If a strain is over 10 percent THC, add 70 extra milligrams for each additional percentage point. For example, if a strain is 11% THC and you infuse 1 cup of butter with 7 grams of cannabis, it will be 770 milligrams of THC total in the entire batch. Similarly, you would wind up with 840 milligrams for a 12% strain, 1050 milligrams for a 15% strain, and so on. If your preferred cannabis strain is CBD dominant, use the same calculations above to reflect amounts of CBD in your infusion.

If you find that after testing, the batch of weed butter or oil you made was too weak for your preference, feel free to increase the grams of weed by increments of 7 to more easily calculate potency. For example, if the standard dose of 14 grams (½ ounce) is too low for you, but you don't want to add an entire ounce, just increase the amount of weed you're using by 7 grams for a total of 21 grams of cannabis—that's ¾ ounce.

If you find that the batch is too strong, dilute your batch by adding one additional cup of butter, oil, or fat to your infusion, and mix evenly by shaking and stirring. Once it is cooled, try one teaspoon of the new mix and see how your body feels.

Storage

You know this one: Store in a cool, dry, and dark place. Pretty standard, right? Be sure to contain your weed butter and cannabis-infused oils and fats in a tightly sealed container or jar. I suggest glass jars with metal or plastic lids. Because your butter, oil, or fat is infused with cannabis, there is a chance that the potency of the infusion might degrade after two to three months, degrading more each time the container is exposed to air, sun, or light. And, as always, please keep your infusions out of the reach of children or pets. Here are some more specific storage tips:

Cannabutter: Well-sealed mason jar or container. Lasts up to six months refrigerated or frozen.

Cannabis Oil: Well-sealed mason jar or container. Lasts up to one year.

Cannabis Fats: Keep in a well-sealed mason jar. Can last from one to three months.

Infusing Cannabis

As it turns out, there are a million ways to extract the healing properties of weed into oil, butter, or fat. But it's important to find a method that works best for you. You don't have to be a master chef or cannabis connoisseur to make great weed butter. You just need to be well-informed, patient, and organized. Most folks who are looking to make edibles are patients or people who want to medicate independently, discreetly, and inexpensively.

We're all just everyday folks looking for an efficient way to get high, so don't feel daunted by this at all.

Decarboxylation

The first thing you'll have to do, regardless of which method you're using, is decarboxylate your cannabis material. Also known as "decarbing," this requires you to bake your weed, allowing the THC or CBD to activate.

Raw, unsmoked cannabis contains various cannabinoids, including THCA and CBDA. These cannabinoids need to be heated in order to turn into THC or CBD. This happens when you smoke a joint, for example. It's an instant decarboxylation that helps you to achieve your high. THCA is great for you too, but it won't give you the same effects as THC. Decarbing is a necessary step in order to enjoy the full spectrum of the cannabis you consume. Also, it allows for the lipids (such as fatty acids, waxes, and some vitamins) in the butter or oils to easily bind to your weed for the ultimate cannabis infusion.

Though you can use top-notch, beautiful cannabis flowers from your local dispensary, feel free to use trimmings, stems, and/or stalks. If you're someone who cultivates weed, it's a great way to cut back on waste while using the entire plant. Just be sure that the quality of the plant is clean (free of pesticides, mold, etc.) and that the material is frosty with some trichomes.

WHAT YOU'LL NEED

desired amount of weed (¼ ounce, ½ ounce, or 1 ounce) hand grinder or scissors

glass baking dish or sheet pan

oven

WHAT TO DO

1. Preheat the oven to 220°F.

2. Gently break apart the desired amount of weed using a hand-grinder,

scissors, or with hands until it's the perfect consistency for rolling a joint—

fine, but not too fine. Anything too fine will slip through cheesecloth (or a

joint, for that matter). You want your cannabutter and oil to be clean and as

clear as possible.

3. Evenly spread your plant material onto the glass baking dish or sheet pan.

Pop in the oven on the center rack for 20 minutes if using old or lower

quality weed; 45 minutes for cured, high-grade weed; or 1 hour or more for

anything that has been recently harvested and is still wet.

4. Check on the weed frequently while it's in the oven, gently mixing it

every 10 minutes so as to not burn it. You will notice that the color of your herb will change from bright green to a deep brownish green. That's when you know it has decarboxylated.

Just so you know, while you're decarbing, your kitchen will smell like one giant edible. I love the way it smells, personally. But if

you're worried about neighbors, close windows and burn incense, palo santo, sage, candles, or whatever you prefer. Another great idea is to cook or bake something while your weed is decarbing. The other aromas will fill your home as well.

Clarified Butter

Though not absolutely important, clarifying butter beforehand can result in a more even consistency of weed butter. Similar to ghee, clarified butter is butterfat that has been separated from milk solids and water.

WHAT YOU'LL NEED

8–16 ounces butter

saucepan

mason jar or air-tight container

spoon

1. In a medium saucepan, heat your butter over medium-low heat until it

melts.

2. Once it's fully melted into a liquid, gently skim the white milk solids and any water from the top of the butter with a spoon. Use in your infused cannabutter recipe, or transfer clarified butter into a mason jar or airtight container for later use.

Infusion with Alcohol

1 ounce grain alcohol

½ ounce decarboxylated cannabis material

spray bottle or shot glass and spoon

8 ounces clarified butter, melted butter, oil, or fat

slow cooker

spoon

cheesecloth

storage container of choice

1. Pour 1 ounce of grain alcohol directly onto your decarboxylated marijuana. You can use a spray bottle to evenly distribute the alcohol among the decarbed cannabis, or you can use a 1-ounce shot glass and small spoon.

Suggested Additional Infusion Herbs and Roots

When infusing weed, especially with the slow cooker and sous vide

method, you can add an herb or root of choice if you're looking for

some added flavor profiles. Here are a few I like to include during

infusion (individually, or paired to your liking).

• Basil

• Cilantro

• Chives

• Garlic

• Ginger

• Mint

• Oregano

• Peppercorns

• Turmeric

Simply add a desired amount of herbs or roots to your butter before

you begin the infusion process, and strain them out when you strain

the weed.

Cannabutters

Classic Cannabutter

Butter has a bad rap and weed butter has swooped in to save its name.

Despite having been demonized in the past, butter (especially from grassfed cows) is actually pretty healthy. Cannabutter, a.k.a. weed butter, can go with almost everything, but I find that it complements baked goods, pastas, and rice dishes the best. Use a little or as much as you want to get the kind of relief or experience you desire.

Vegan Cannabutter, Margarine, and Ghee

Use vegan weed butter and margarine the same as you would regular butter.

Add a slab onto pancakes, or even rice, for a creamier and more complex flavor. Ghee, essentially clarified butter, is in a class of its

own. It's been recently hyped up by Westerners for its nuttier flavor—this is after 30 years of shaming it for its high fat contents. Ghee, originally from the Indian subcontinent, loosely translates to "sprinkle" in Sanskrit. So sprinkle, or spread, it on anything you want, or anything that calls for butter.

And since ghee separates milk from fat, it's essentially lactose-free, making it better than butter if you have to avoid dairy products. Cannabis-Infused Sunflower, Grapeseed, and

Canola Oils

Sunflower oil is the high-heat priestess, with a super-high smoking point of 440°F. It's followed by grapeseed oil at 420°F (this is a coincidence), and canola at a cool 400°F—which isn't cool at all. These types of oils are perfect to use for stir fries and fried dishes. Sunflower oil contains a small amount of pollen, which boosts its nutritional and THC-binding qualities.

Cannabis-Infused Coconut Oil

I love coconut oil. I use it topically on my skin and I cook with it. With nearly 86 percent of it containing healthy saturated fats, it's both a healthy and vegan option. Coconut oil has a burning point of about 350°F, so feel

free to sauté with it, but do not fry with it. Swap it for butter in sweet or

savory dishes. It's great for soups, stews, and baking.

Cannabis-Infused Avocado Seed Oil

Like the oil of the gods, goddesses, and other deities, avocado seed oil cures

everything with a luxurious edge. Drizzle cannabis-infused avocado oil on

toast, rice, or fish. Use it on your face for sun damage, psoriasis, or acne.

Slather it on your hair as a hot-oil treatment to deeply moisturize afros and

locks. Unrefined, cold-pressed, extravirgin avocado oil is best, as it's known

to be packed with vitamins B and C and to contribute to the prevention of

heart disease and cancer.

Cannabis-Infused Olive Oil

Olive oil has made its way into our hearts and bellies for centuries. It's the

best canna oil for salad dressings, drizzling over soups (hot and cold),

prepared food, pasta, sauces, or even your skin. It's exceptionally high in

oleic acid, which is known to burn fat, assist with weight loss, and help

reduce high blood pressure. Olive oil also contains many antioxidants,

including vitamin E, carotenoids, and oleuropein.

Low-Dose
Breakfasts

Morning Medicated Fruit Bowl

This medicated fruit

bowl is healthy, pretty, and easy to make. Use any berries you'd like, such

as strawberries, blueberries, raspberries, or blackberries. What's more, it's packed with enough energy to keep you full and focused throughout the

morning, with a healthy dose of THC to chill you the *bleep* out before

tackling a potentially stressful day.

Time: 5 minutes Potency per serving: 15 mg Yield: 2 servings

WHAT YOU'LL NEED

1½ cups plain yogurt

1 teaspoon cannabis-infused coconut oil, or as desired

1 tablespoon chia seeds, nuts, or granola

1 handful berries

½ banana, sliced, optional

WHAT TO DO

1. Spoon out your yogurt into a bowl, mason jar, or large cup. Add your

desired amount of cannabis-infused coconut oil.

2. Whip gently with a spoon or fork until evenly mixed. Mix in any seeds,

nuts, or granola.

3. Top with berries and banana, if using, and enjoy!

Easy Cheese Cannabis Spinach Frittata

The word "frittata" always seems fancy, but really, it's just a large omelet

that you never have to flip—or is it a quiche without a pie crust? Either

way, it's one of the simplest breakfast dishes that can "wow" anyone. Feel

free to stick to the recipe and use the ingredients below, or add whatever

vegetables or cheeses that are already hanging out in your refrigerator.

Time: 25 minutes Potency per serving: 3 mg Yield: 5 servings

WHAT YOU'LL NEED

½ medium onion, diced

2 cloves garlic, minced

2 tablespoons olive oil

1 cup spinach or other leafy greens

5 eggs

½ cup milk, dairy or nondairy

1 small tomato, sliced

1 teaspoon cannabutter or cannabis-infused olive oil

½ cup grated melting cheese

salt and black pepper, to taste

WHAT TO DO

1. In a medium pan over medium heat, sauté the onion and garlic in olive

oil for 5 minutes, letting them cook until transparent and your kitchen

smells like heaven.

2. Add cannabutter or cannabis-infused olive oil and spinach or other green

leafy vegetables and cook for 1 to 2 minutes.

3. Whisk the eggs with milk and pour evenly over the veggies.

4. Spread the cheese over the eggs like it's a pizza, placing the sliced

tomatoes similarly.

5. Cover the eggs with a lid or plate for 5 to 10 minutes on low heat, or

longer if you like your eggs extra crispy at the bottom. The eggs will puff

up, signifying that they're done.

6. Remove the lid, slice into six slices, and enjoy!

Simple Stoney Hash Browns

Time: 30 minutes Potency per serving: 7.25 mg Yield: 2 servings

WHAT YOU'LL NEED

1 pound (about 3 large) potatoes

3 tablespoons extra-virgin olive oil

1 teaspoon cannabis-infused olive oil or cannabutter

salt and black pepper, to taste

WHAT TO DO

1. Shred the potatoes with a cheese grater. Be careful with your fingers. The

bigger the potatoes you use, the better. Once grated, season with salt and

pepper, to taste.

2. Add the olive oil and cannabis-infused olive oil or cannabutter to a

medium pan or skillet over medium heat.

3. Add the shredded potatoes evenly and let them cook until you see the

bottom start to become crisp, about 8 minutes.

4. Flip with a spatula. (The skillet should be greasy enough for you to do a

pan flip if you wanted—trust me!)

5. Let cook for about 5 minutes, until the hash browns have reached

preferred crispiness.

Sauces, Spreads, and Dressings

Canna-oil Chocolate Hazelnut Spread

Eat a spoonful to curb

your stoned sweet tooth. Spread it on toast, add it to a smoothie, or use it as

a frosting on cake, brownies. Melt it on strawberries, blackberries, bananas

—any fruit of choice. This is super easy to make, which means you get to

put it in your mouth that much sooner.

Time: 2 minutes Potency per tablespoon: 1 mg Yield: 24 tablespoons

(1½ cups)

WHAT YOU'LL NEED

1 (375-gram) jar of Nutella or another store-bought chocolate hazelnut

spread

2 tablespoons cannabutter or cannabis-infused coconut oil

WHAT TO DO

Add the cannabis-infused coconut oil or weed butter to Nutella. Mix well

by hand. Serve and enjoy.

Philly Jalapeño Crema

Time: 20 minutes Potency per recipe: 14.5 mg Yield: 2 cups

WHAT YOU'LL NEED

6 jalapeños

½ bunch of cilantro

1 tablespoon olive oil

1 teaspoon cannabis-infused olive oil

1 tablespoon cumin

pinch of cayenne

3 to 5 cloves garlic, minced

salt and black pepper, to taste

WHAT TO DO

1. Add the jalapeños to a small saucepan. Fill with just enough water to

cover. Bring the water to a boil, then lower to a simmer. Cook for about 15

minutes. Drain.

2. In a blender, add the boiled jalapeños, cilantro, both oils, cumin, cayenne,

garlic, salt, and pepper, and blend until it reaches a thick but creamy

consistency. Add more water if necessary.

Elevated Tomato Sauce

The legs of this sauce are the

tomatoes (canned tomatoes are fine), salt, and cannabutter. The rest is up to

you! Serve as a pizza sauce, a dip for breadsticks, a simple pasta sauce, or base for tomato soup.

Time: 1 hour Potency per recipe: 14.5 mg Yield: 3 cups

WHAT YOU'LL NEED

2 cups chopped tomatoes

1 teaspoon cannabutter

2 tablespoons butter

½ teaspoon sugar

2 cloves garlic

1 tablespoon salt

1 tablespoon crushed black pepper

1 tablespoon red pepper flakes

1 cup shredded Parmesan cheese

WHAT DO TO

1. Add all ingredients to a large saucepan and bring to a simmer on low

heat. Be sure to not let the butter burn too fast.

2. Let simmer, covered, for 45 minutes to an hour, stirring and smashing

tomatoes and garlic every 15 minutes. I prefer to keep mine chunky and

rustic. If you fancy a pureed consistency, once cooled, blend the sauce with

a blender or a food processor.

Nutty Vegan Chipotle Aioli

Time: 10 minutes, plus time to soak Potency per recipe: 14.5 mg Yield:

1 cup

WHAT YOU'LL NEED

1 cup raw cashews

½ cup soy, almond, or coconut milk

2 to 3 chipotle peppers

1 teaspoon adobo sauce

1 small clove garlic

2 tablespoons lime juice

1 teaspoon agave nectar or raw sugar

1 teaspoon cannabis-infused avocado seed oil

salt, to taste

WHAT TO DO

1. At least one hour up to one night before, soak your cashews in a bowl of

hot water with a pinch of salt; you can either leave the soaking nuts on your

counter or refrigerate. Strain cashews and store covered in the refrigerator

until ready to blend.

2. In a blender, add the soaked cashews, milk, peppers, adobo sauce, and

garlic, and pulse until smooth.

3. Add the lime, sugar, cannabis-infused oil, and a pinch of salt.

4. Blend until smooth, using a wooden spoon to remove any chunks that

might not be blending.

5. Store in the refrigerator for up to one week.

Classic Weed Balsamic Vinaigrette

Time: 15 minutes Potency per recipe: 30 mg Yield: 1 cup

WHAT YOU'LL NEED

2 cloves garlic, finely chopped

1 teaspoon salt

1 teaspoon ground pepper

1 teaspoon Dijon mustard

1 teaspoon cannabis-infused olive oil

4 tablespoons olive oil

3 tablespoons balsamic vinegar

WHAT TO DO

In a dish, whisk together the garlic pieces, salt, pepper, Dijon, and cannabisinfused

oil. Add the regular olive oil and vinegar and whisk to combine.

Add more vinegar or oil to your taste.

Green Ganja Dressing

Time: 15 minutes Potency per recipe: 30 mg Yield: 2 cups

WHAT YOU'LL NEED

1½ cups plain yogurt

1½ packed cups basil leaves

¼ packed cup chives

2 cloves garlic

1 green onion, chopped

2 anchovy fillets, optional

1 teaspoon lime juice

1 lime, zested

1 tablespoon extra-virgin olive oil

2 teaspoons cannabis-infused olive oil

salt and pepper, to taste

WHAT TO DO

Add all the ingredients into a blender and purée. Add salt and black pepper

to taste.

Guacamole Mágico

Time: 10 minutes Potency per recipe: 14.5 mg Yield: 2 cups

WHAT YOU'LL NEED

4 avocados, pitted

½ small onion, minced

½ jalapeño, minced

1 teaspoon salt

2 cloves garlic, minced

1 teaspoon cannabis-infused olive oil

fresh or dried cilantro, for garnish

WHAT TO DO

Scoop all the avocado flesh into a medium bowl. Add the remaining

ingredients and mix with a spoon to reach your desired chunkiness. Garnish

with cilantro.

Mains and Sides

Cute and Cheesy Macaroni Bake

Time: 45 minutes Potency per serving: 3.75 mg Yield: 4 servings

WHAT YOU'LL NEED

2 cups dry macaroni pasta

2 tablespoons flour

½ cup cream cheese

1 cup milk

1 tablespoon butter, room temperature

1 teaspoon cannabutter, room temperature

½ teaspoon salt

½ teaspoon freshly ground black pepper

pinch red pepper flakes

3 cloves garlic, minced

1½ cups shredded white cheddar cheese, divided

WHAT TO DO

1. Preheat the oven to 375°F.

2. In a medium pot, boil water. Once boiling, add the macaroni.

3. Cook pasta on medium-high heat for 7 to 10 minutes, or until al dente,

then strain.

4. Put strained pasta into a large mixing bowl, then add the flour, cream

cheese, milk, butters, salt, pepper, red pepper flakes, garlic, and half of the

cheddar. Mix well to combine.

5. Transfer the pasta mixture into four individual oven-safe ramekins or, if

you'd prefer, an oven-safe baking dish. Then, add the remaining cheddar on

top.

6. Bake for 20 minutes until the cheese is bubbly and slightly browned.

7. Let sit for 5 minutes to cool before serving.

West African Fried Chicken

Time: 50 minutes, plus time to marinate Potency per piece: 3.75 mg

Yield: 8 pieces

WHAT YOU'LL NEED

3 pounds (8 mixed pieces) chicken

2 teaspoons cannabis-infused grapeseed oil

2 teaspoons salt

2 teaspoons black pepper

2 large cloves garlic, finely chopped

1 to 2 tablespoons chopped serrano or jalapeño peppers

1 teaspoon honey

1 egg

½ cup milk

2 cups flour

1 tablespoon cornmeal (grits or polenta)

vegetable oil, for frying

WHAT TO DO

1. Clean the chicken and pat dry, then place it in a large bowl. Add the

cannabis-infused grapeseed oil into the bowl. Stir with a wooden spoon or

wooden spatula to make sure the oil coats the chicken evenly. This will

ensure the most accurate dose per piece.

2. Add salt, black pepper, garlic, hot peppers, and honey, continuing to stir

until the chicken is coated evenly.

3. Place chicken in the refrigerator for at least 10 minutes to overnight.

4. In a medium bowl, whisk the egg and milk together. In a separate bowl,

sift the flour and cornmeal together.

5. Remove the marinated chicken from refrigerator.

6. In a deep frying pan, add about 1 inch of vegetable oil. Turn the burner

up to medium-high heat. Allow the oil to heat up for 1 or 2 minutes. To test the heat, sprinkle a tiny grain of your flour mixture. If it pops up to surface,

it's ready for your chicken.

7. Dip each piece of chicken into the whisked egg and milk mixture, then

into the flour. Gently pat the flour onto the chicken so that it sticks and

coats each piece. Gently place the chicken pieces into the frying pan. Make

sure to leave a little space in between each piece to keep them from sticking

together while frying.

8. With tongs or a large metal spoon, turn each piece every 5 minutes for

about 20 minutes total, until the pieces are perfectly brown. If it seems like

the chicken is cooking too fast or spattering too much oil, turn the burner

down to medium.

9. Once cooked, place the chicken onto a couple sheets of wax paper or

paper towels. Let rest for a couple minutes and then serve

Garlic-Crunch Sweet Potato Fries

They have obscene amounts of potassium, vitamin C, fiber, and

calcium, and are known by some health gurus to help fight cancer because

of their antioxidant properties. Sweet potatoes help lower blood sugar,

despite being sweet. They're also a great, inexpensive baby food. Just bake

in the oven in aluminum foil and mash up for the baby. She'll love them!

But this recipe is not for babies—it's just for fancy grown-ups at a weedinfused

dinner.

Time: 45 minutes Potency per serving: 3.75 mg Yield: 4 servings

WHAT YOU'LL NEED

3 medium sweet potatoes, peeled as desired, cut lengthwise into ½-inch

strips

2 large cloves garlic, minced

pinch of coarse salt

1 teaspoon crushed black pepper

pinch of cayenne

4 tablespoons coconut oil

1 teaspoon cannabis-infused sunflower oil

WHAT TO DO

1. Preheat the oven to 400°F.

2. Place the potatoes in a baking dish, spreading them out evenly.

3. Mix in your spices and oils, making sure to coat the potatoes evenly.

Bake for 45 minutes, until crispy. Mix halfway through the cooking time.

CONCLUSION

Food infused with cannabis has a long association with healing both the body and mind. The types of food we take in, especially superfoods, can help fill the void of what our body is lacking and craving in order to thrive. Nutritionally dense foods, or superfoods (cleverly named by marketers) like broccoli, blueberries, and leafy greens are absorbed to fortify our body with vitamins and nutrients. Cannabis, and by extension tetrahydrocannabinol

(THC), could also be considered a superfood.

THC is what most people think of when they think of weed. It gives you the

euphoric "high" effects, and can also affect the way you feel pain, hunger, and moods. It can help with inflammation, nausea, and nerve pain, and help increase appetites. No wonder it's used as a treatment for all types of diseases.

Cannabis as an entire plant is the multipurpose food of all foods. We can juice its leaves or grind the seeds to put in smoothies and baked goods. We can use its stalks to make rope, bricks, fuel, cloth, and paper. We dry its flowers to smoke, vape, or create oils to eat or apply directly onto our skin.